A

Guide To Healing Fibroids And Ovarian Cyst Naturally

7 Herbal Remedies I Used To Heal My Fibroid Tumors And Ovarian Cyst At Home

FAVOUR MARIUS

DEDICATION

This book is dedicated to the Almighty God of creation, who gave this insight and granted me healing using these herbs.

And also to my fiancé who stood by me throughout my time of trial.

TABLE OF CONTENT

DEDICATION

TABLE OF CONTENT

DISCLAIMER

HOW TO USE THIS BOOK

CHAPTER ONE
  WHAT IS FIBROID?
  WHY CAUSES UTERINE FIBROIDS TO GROW?
  DO FIBROIDS HAVE SYMPTOMS OR SIGNS?
  TYPES OF FIBROIDS
  HOW DO I KNOW IF I HAVE FIBROIDS OR CYSTS?
  WHAT YOU SHOULD KNOW ABOUT FIBROIDS?
  CAN FIBROID OR OVARIAN CYSTS GO AWAY ON THEIR OWN
  WHAT IS THE BEST TREATMENT FOR FIBROID?

CHAPTER TWO
  WHY ARE YOUR FIBROIDS NOT GOING AWAY?
  WHAT YOU ARE DOING WRONG?
  FOODS TO AVOID WHEN TRYING TO SHRINK FIBROIDS NATURALLY
  FOODS YOU CAN EAT WHEN YOU'RE TRYING TO SHRINK FIBROIDS NATURALLY
  DETOXIFY YOUR BODY AS AT WHEN NEEDED
  21 HERBAL TEAS THAT WILL SHRINK YOUR FIBROIDS AND OVARIAN CYSTS
  12 KEY SUCCESSES TO SHRINK FIBROIDS AND OVARIAN CYSTS

CHAPTER THREE
  MY FIBROID AND CYSTS JOURNEY STORY

CHAPTER FOUR
  SEVEN HERBAL SOLUTIONS FOR HEALING FIBROIDS AND OVARIAN CYSTS

CHAPTER FIVE
  SMOOTHIES AND JUICES FOR HEALING FIBROIDS AND OVARIAN CYSTS
  NATURAL DRINKS FOR HEALING FIBROIDS AND OVARIAN CYSTS
  ANTI INFLAMMATORY TEAS AND SMOOTHIES
  POWERFUL HORMONE BALANCING SMOOTHIES

HERBS IMAGES FOR EASY RECOGNITION

DISCLAIMER

This information is not presented by a medical practitioner and is for educational and informational purposes only.

The content is not intended to be a substitute for professional medical advice, diagnosis, or treatment.

Always seek the advice of your physician or other qualified health provider with any questions you may have regarding a medical condition.

Never disregard professional medical advice or delay in seeking it because of something you have read.

Since natural and/or dietary supplements are not FDA approved they must be accompanied by a two part disclaimer on the product label:

That the statement on this book has not been evaluated by FDA and that the product is not intended to "diagnose, treat, cure or prevent any disease."

I do not in any way guarantee you that you will get the exact result that I got because of our body differences.

No two people have the same body system. What worked for me may not work for you and what worked for you may not work for me.

Just give it a try. It may be the solution you're looking for.

Note

If you're using these remedies and you want to get results with it, YOU MUST AVOID EVERYTHING YOU ARE TOLD NOT TO EAT in this book.

Secondly, you must be consistent with the remedies, DRINK and EAT HEALTHY.

HOW TO USE THIS BOOK

In chapter four of this book, I have listed the seven herbal solutions I used in 2021 to get rid of my fibroid and ovarian cysts.

Few of these herbs like Aidan fruit (Tetrapleura Tetrapetra), piper guineense, etc. are particular to Africa but can be found online in any part of the world where you're. You can always buy them from online malls like Amazon, Walmart, even your local malls etc. whereas others like cloves, ginger, cinnamon etc. are common round the world.

I have added the images of these herbs at the last pages of this book to help you easily recognize or identify them.

There are 7 herbal solutions to prepare directly from your kitchen. You don't need a third party to help you.

All you have to do is to get the herbs from the market, wash them and prepare them as directed.

You're to use the remedies as follows: one month, one remedy. You should use one remedy for a whole month before you change to another remedy if you wish to or rather stick to one remedy until you're totally healed.

These herbal remedies/solutions can be used by anyone (woman) that has fibroids, ovarian cysts, irregular menstrual flow/ovulation, yeast or bacterial infections, blocked fallopian tube, PCOS, or any other female related diseases.

Aside from healing the fibroid and cysts, remedy number six can be taken by men and women experiencing delay in conception due to hormonal imbalance.

Number one to number five herbal solutions should be taken three times daily (morning on empty stomach 1 hour before breakfast, 2 hours before lunch, and last thing to bed at night. **And the remedies must be taken when it's still hot.**

The remedy number six and number seven should be taken ½ glass twice daily not three times because it aids weight loss and belly fat loss.

So if you're skinny like me, don't use these remedies more than once in a month if not you'll look for yourself. The two remedies will be best for those who want to lose weight. But they're good at healing ovarian cysts.

While taking these herbal remedies, remember they are herbs so don't expect immediate healing. Herbs work slowly, you'll have to take these remedies for like 90 to 365 days before you could receive total healing depending on the size of your fibroids or cysts.

Finally I pray for your quick recovery as I have recovered. Good luck.

CHAPTER ONE

Fact number 1: By the time they reach menopause, forty percent of American women have at least one uterine fibroid; 600,000 women are diagnosed each year.

Fact number 2: Fibroids are the leading cause of hysterectomy, the second most common surgical procedure performed on women.

Fact number 3: 30–77% of women have or will suffer uterine fibroids, and about 30% of those women are of reproductive age. Yet there is no medical solution for it except surgery.

Fact number 4: Research shows that Black women (i.e Africa) are more likely to develop fibroids.

Fact number 5: Research also shows that fibroids usually develop at a younger age, grow faster and bigger, and cause more severe symptoms for Black women.

Fact number 6: They're most common for people ages 30-40.

Fact number 7: Natural, holistic medicine can heal fibroids without invasive surgery.

WHAT IS FIBROID?

Uterine fibroids also known as uterine leiomyomas or myomas are muscle growth (tumor) either inside or outside of the uterus (womb).

They are not cancerous at all in any way but can cause lots of damage to the person having it.

For example, fibroids can cause you heavy bleeding during your menstrual flow and/or even when not in menstrual flows, fibroids can also cause miscarriage and infertility in women of childbearing age, especially those ones that grow inside the uterus.

Therefore, it's not safe to keep these fibroids with you as long as you're still the childbearing age, except you don't want to have your own children.

WHAT CAUSES UTERINE FIBROIDS TO GROW?

No one actually knows the causes of fibroids. No researchers or medical experts have been able to discover the causes of Fibroids and Ovarian Cysts.

However, there are risk factors that may trigger the growth of fibroids in the uterus and ovarian cysts in the ovaries.

The main risk factor of uterine fibroids and ovarian cyst is **Hormonal Imbalance.**

As a woman you have two dominant hormones in your system that control fertility and menstrual cycles, which are progesterone and estrogen.

One specific hormone that needs to be controlled in life is **estrogen.** Women with estrogen dominance are particularly at the risk of developing fibroids and ovarian cyst, also in order to control existing fibroids from getting bigger, balancing the hormone level is critical.

This simply means that your estrogen hormone and progesterone hormone must be balanced if you want to be free from fibroids and the related diseases.

So Uterine Fibroids are linked to excess estrogen in the body, a condition called Estrogen Dominance.

Estrogen Dominance (or ED) is a term that describes a condition where a woman can have deficient, normal or excessive estrogen, but has little or no progesterone to balance its effects in her body.

Even a woman with low estrogen levels can have estrogen dominance symptoms if she doesn't have enough progesterone in her body to balance it out.

Uterine Fibroids grow when the liver cannot metabolize all the excess estrogen in the body or if your body can't eliminate the estrogen through the body's five elimination channels.

Therefore, the estrogen gets stored in the fat cells (weight gain) and other weak parts of the body such as the uterus and the breasts. Too much estrogen can cause your uterus to grow excessively.

Ultimately, Uterine Fibroids grow because of what we eat and drink, our emotional, mental and spiritual status, environmental factors i.e. what we put on our bodies (lotions, hair products, makeup), vitamin and mineral deficiencies, and more.

All of these factors can cause estrogen dominance and cause Uterine Fibroids to develop and grow.

Other Risk Factors Includes:

1. Family history of uterine fibroid (especially your mother)
2. If you're are obese (obesity)
3. If you eat lots of red meat
4. If you don't get enough vitamin D
5. Someone that had an early onset of menstruation (getting your period at a young age).
6. Someone that entered menopause late.
7. High blood pressure
8. No history of pregnancy
9. Food additive consumption
10. Use of soybean milk or soy products
11. Pregnancy (the risk decreases with an increasing number of pregnancies)
12. Long-term use of oral or injectable contraceptives

DO FIBROIDS HAVE SYMPTOMS?

Uterine fibroids don't always cause symptoms. Around 1 in 3 women with fibroids will experience symptoms. If you do have symptoms of uterine fibroids, they can include:

- Longer or heavier periods
- Bleeding between periods
- Painful cramp
- Anemia (from losing too much blood during your period)
- Pain in your belly or lower back
- Pain during sex
- Feeling full in the lower part of your belly (called pelvic pressure)
- Swelling in your uterus or belly
- Peeing a lot or having a hard time peeing
- Constipation or pain while pooping
- Miscarriage
- Problems during labor, like being more likely to have a cesarean section
- Infertility (this is rare and can often be treated)

The size of your fibroids isn't related to how bad your symptoms are. Even small fibroids can cause problems.

TYPES OF FIBROIDS

There are several places both inside and outside of your uterus where fibroids can grow. The location and size of your fibroids is important for your treatment.

Where your fibroids are growing, how big they are and how many of them you have will determine which type of treatment will work best for you or if treatment is even necessary.

There are different names given for the places your fibroids are located in and on the uterus. These names describe not only where the fibroid is, but how it's attached. Specific locations where you can have uterine fibroids include:

1.   **Submucosal Fibroids**

In this case, the fibroids are growing inside the uterine space (cavity) where a baby grows during pregnancy. Think of the growths extending down into the empty space in the middle of the uterus.

2.   **Intramural Fibroids**

These fibroids are embedded into the wall of the uterus itself. Picture the sides of the uterus like walls of a house. The fibroids are growing inside this muscular wall. This is the one I had.

3.   **Subserosal Fibroids**

It's located on the outside of the uterus this time. These fibroids are connected closely to the outside wall of the uterus.

4.   **Pedunculated Fibroids**

The least common type, these fibroids are also located on the outside of the uterus. However, pedunculated fibroids are connected to the uterus with a thin stem. They're often described as mushroom-like because they have a stalk and then a much wider top.

HOW DO I KNOW IF I HAVE FIBROIDS OR CYSTS?

Once you started having any type of pelvic or lower abdomen pain. My dear, run to the hospital immediately, your doctor or Sonographer will carry out any of these tests to see if you have fibroids or cysts.

They may use ultrasounds, X-rays, MRIs, CAT scans, or other types of imaging technology to take a picture of the inside of your body.

Don't say it's ordinary stomach pain or ache. I am speaking to you out of experience. It is better the scan say it's ordinary stomach pain than you saying because by the time the pain will be heavy on you, the fibroid would have grown large.

Herbal treatment of the early fibroid is faster and easier than treatment of large fibroids.

She who has ears should hear now!

WHAT YOU SHOULD KNOW ABOUT FIBROIDS?

- Fibroids are most common during the reproductive years.
- It is unclear exactly why they form, but they appear to develop when estrogen levels are higher.
- Most people experience no symptoms, but they can include lower backache, constipation, and excessive or painful uterine bleeding leading to anemia.
- Complications are rare, but they can be serious.

CAN FIBROID OR OVARIAN CYSTS GO AWAY ON THEIR OWN

Well fibroids can go away when a woman has entered menopause age. That's the age at which progesterone and estrogen hormone has stopped producing. So at this point the fibroids shrink and die away.

But for ovarian cysts, it depends on the type of ovarian cysts you are diagnosed with. If yours is functional cysts, functional cysts often go away on their own after some time.

However, if it is a dermoid, Cystadenomas, Endometriomas, and PCOS, they don't go away or shrink on their own.

You have to either go for surgery to remove them or heal yourself naturally using herbs, spices and foods as medicine just like I did mine.

I will always advise my fellow women to seek healing through herbs and change of diets because this method of healing is best because it heals both the problem and the cause of the problem.

Surgery only removes the problem and not the cause of the problem. So there is every tendency that fibroids and cysts would always grow again after surgery because the causes are still there.

WHAT IS THE BEST TREATMENT FOR FIBROID?

Your medical treatment for uterine fibroids will depend on: your age, your general health, how bad your symptoms are, the size, type, and location of your fibroids and whether you want to get pregnant in the future

However, your doctor can give you some medicine to manage the pain or you may require surgery, or you can use herbs and spices like I did.

Healing yourself with herbs is the ultimate but bear it in mind that healing through herbs will take time so you need to be patient and determined. Otherwise you can opt for surgery that's a quick fix.

Why I love healing with herbs is because herbs heal both the root cause of the problem and the problem itself.

But if you go for surgery, the Surgeon will only remove the problem (fibroids), not the causes, the reason why people who have gone for surgery will go for second surgery even third surgery because the causes are still there.

I so much believed in herbs. I used it and it worked for me. Those exact remedies that I used to get a positive result, is what I will be sharing with you in this book.

CHAPTER TWO

WHY ARE YOUR FIBROIDS NOT GOING AWAY?

I have heard many women saying that shrinking fibroids naturally through herbs is not possible. When I hear such comments from women I always laugh because they don't understand the tricks.

Healing fibroids using foods and herbs as medicine is very possible. I did it and it worked for me. The only thing is that there are rules you must follow very strictly if you actually prefer healing yourself with herbs and foods.

Many women had tried herbal remedies/home remedies in the past to shrink their fibroid and it didn't yield results. That doesn't mean that natural remedies are not working but there is something they didn't do right.

And that's what I want to address in this chapter of this book.

WHAT YOU ARE DOING WRONG?

So many things you're doing wrong. No matter the type of herbal remedy you are giving, if you don't strictly follow the rules that follow that remedy strictly, you won't get results.

If you're drinking herbal remedies and you're still eating those foods that trigger fibroid growth and even increase their size, you're making a dangerous mistake because you're just feeding the fibroids to keep growing bigger and not to shrink it.

Herbal remedies will shrink fibroids and cysts if you avoid those foods and items that make fibroids thrive in the uterus, rather feed yourself on those foods that will starve them and cause the fibroids to die natural death without resurrection.

Below is the list of foods to avoid when you're drinking any natural remedies to shrink your fibroids or ovarian cyst.

FOODS TO AVOID WHEN TRYING TO SHRINK FIBROIDS NATURALLY

The foods and/or food categories listed below contribute to Uterine Fibroids. This is NOT an exhaustive list but it will get you started on your journey to health. Food is the major contributor to fibroid.

Sugar – White processed sugar or cane sugar. It is a hormone disruptor, toxic, acidic, inflammatory, and addictive. White sugar contains chemicals as it is bleached to make it white in color. Sugar causes fibroids to grow.

Beverages Containing Caffeine – Especially coffee, black tea, green tea, energy drinks, soda. Usually, caffeine is in foods or products that are hormone disruptors, acidic, and that causes inflammation in the body. The other big problem with caffeine is that it can block the body's ability to absorb iron.

Saturated Fat - Fat from animals, lard and cream, tallow, butter, cheese, ghee. It is acid-forming, mucus forming, a hormone disruptor, toxic, carcinogenic, and causes fibroids to grow.

Processed Foods - Cookies, cakes, chips, candy, bread, crackers, boxed mac n cheese,noodle dishes, flavored rice, biscuits, cereals, etc. Women with fibroids have a digestive system that is backed up and congested. Fibroids wouldn't be present if this wasn't the case and these foods just keep making things worse.

Processed foods are filled with chemicals to make them feel and taste good. Processed food is a chemistry experiment. It is not food. They are boxes, bags, and jars of toxic waste. They are acid-forming, mucus forming, hormone-disruptors, toxic, carcinogenic, and they cause fibroids to grow.

White Foods – Rice, flour, bread, pasta, cakes, cookies, rice cakes, sweets, candies. These white foods are hard on the digestive system and keep it backed up and congested. These foods are devoid of nutrition. You are not getting vitamins and minerals from eating these foods. All you are getting is a full belly.

They are acid forming, mucus forming, hormone-disruptors, toxic, carcinogenic, and cause fibroids to grow.

Processed Meats – Bologna, hot dogs, sausages, smoked meat, beef jerky, canned meat, bacon, ham, and salami. Any meat that has been cured, salted, smoked, dried, orcanned. It is acid-forming, mucus forming, a hormone-disruptor, toxic, carcinogenic,and causes fibroids to grow.

High Fat Dairy Products – Milk, cheese, butter, yogurt, ice cream, sour cream, kefir, etc. -These products are often high in added hormones. Dairy is the worst for fibroids. Dairy is puss from the animal. We don't need milk for vitamin d or calcium.

It is acid-forming, mucus forming, a hormone disruptor, toxic, carcinogenic, and causes fibroids to grow. If you don't eliminate anything else, please eliminate this. It is horrible for your health.

Feedlot Meats – Factory Farms Animal Products – Chicken, pork, beef, turkey, goat, lamb, etc. Any food with a face or a mother is considered an animal product. They are loaded with estrogen and/or estrogen-mimicking chemicals.

They inject and feed these animals with chemicals so that they can keep them healthy enough to sell. They are acid-forming, mucus forming, a hormone disruptor, toxic, carcinogenic, and causes fibroids to grow.

Farm-Raised Fish – avoid all fish and shellfish for best results. I don't recommend eating any fish until you are well and then eat it in moderation or you may choose not to eat it again. People think that fish is better than eating steak. You are sadly mistaken. They have the same impact on your reproductive system. They are acid-forming, mucus forming, a hormone disruptor, toxic, carcinogenic, and cause fibroids to grow according to Chelsea.

Soda and Pasteurized Juices and Juice Concentrates with Sugar Added – These are juices that come in the plastic bottle in the grocery stores like Welches, Hawaiianpunch, Kool-aid, powdered drink mixes, gatorade. It's basically sugar water with preservatives, chemicals, artificial flavoring, added sugar, coloring's high fructose corn syrup, etc.

These drinks are a chemistry experiment. It is not meant to quench your thirst. It is poison. It is acid-forming, mucus forming, a hormone disruptor,toxic, carcinogenic, and causes fibroids to grow.

Soy Foods - Soy Milk, Soy Sauce, Soybeans, Tofu, Edamame - Even the organic varieties. Soy is a heavily sprayed crop and a heavy genetically modified crop which means chemicals. It is acid-forming, mucus forming, a hormone-disruptor, toxic,carcinogenic, and causes fibroids to grow.

Fried Foods - Don't cook your food in oil. Don't eat fried food. It clogs up the body and keeps you from healing. It is acid-forming, mucus forming, a hormone disruptor, toxic, carcinogenic, and causes fibroids to grow.

GMO Foods - Genetically Modified Foods. Some examples of GMO foods are canola oil, corn (popcorn), soy, wheat, peas, tomatoes. GMO foods are a chemistry experiment. It is poisonous because they use chemicals to change the genetic makeup of the food to make it intolerant to pests, last longer, and grow bigger. They are acid-forming, mucus forming, a hormone disruptor, toxic, carcinogenic, and causes fibroids to grow.

Corn - Say not to corn. Even organic. It is a heavily sprayed crop and also a big GMO Food which makes it a chemistry experiment. Corn is hard on digestion. Popcorn turns to goo in the digestive tract and some people can't digest it. It is acid-forming, mucus forming, a hormone disruptor, toxic, carcinogenic, and causes fibroids to grow.

Fat-Free Foods - Fat-Free Foods - Avoid packaged foods that say they are fat-free. They are loaded with sugar and chemicals. A poison concoction of chemicals. It is acid-forming, mucus forming, a hormone disruptor, toxic, carcinogenic, and causes fibroids to grow.

Artificial Sweeteners - Avoid Equal, Splenda, Sweet n Low. They are loaded with sugar and chemicals. A poison concoction of chemicals. It is not food. It is also very addictive. It is acid-forming, mucus forming, a hormone disruptor, toxic, carcinogenic, and causes fibroids to grow.

Grains – Avoiding all grains for best results - rice, flour, wheat, bread, pasta - Use quinoa (technically a seed) sparingly if necessary. It is not good for digestion and they contribute to bleeding, pain, and slow the healing process. Grains create mucus, inflammation, and can disrupt hormones.

Alcohol – Turns into sugar which causes uterine fibroids to grow. It is a hormone disruptor, causing estrogen dominance. It causes inflammation in the body. It is addictive like cocaine, acid-forming, mucus forming, a hormone disruptor, toxic, carcinogenic, and causes fibroids to grow.

Fast Food – Usually the food is processed or filled with chemicals. Fast food is fake food. Don't eat it. You are not getting any nutrients from it. It is acid-forming, mucus forming, a hormone disruptor, toxic, carcinogenic, and causes fibroids to grow.

Plastic Bottles - Don't drink water out of plastic bottles. They contain BPA. A chemical that causes fibroids to grow. If you must drink out of plastic containers be sure it is BPA-free. A few brands that are BPA-free are Smart Water, Essentia, Fiji. It is acid-forming, mucus forming, a hormone disruptor, toxic, carcinogenic, and causes fibroids to grow.

Table Salt – It is loaded with chemicals such as bleach. Just because it is labeled as seasalt, it doesn't mean it is healthy. Use Himalayan or Celtic salt instead. It is acid-forming, mucus forming, a hormone disruptor, toxic, carcinogenic, and causes fibroids to grow

Gluten-Free Foods - Don't eat foods marketed as gluten-free i.e. bread, crackers, cookies, etc. – What you get when you eat gluten-free foods is potato starch, cornstarch, and any other starch that makes food taste good without the gluten. The problem is, all those starches are equally bad for you, or a close second and they can make fibroids grow.

Coffee - Don't drink coffee. It is acidic. When trying to heal you want to eat foods that are more on the alkaline side of chemistry. It is acid-forming, mucus forming, inflammatory, and toxic for women with reproductive issues.

Oils (ALL) - STOP cooking with ALL oils and do not pour oil on your food if you want to shrink fibroids naturally. Don't even saute your veggies in oil. Use vegetable broth, coco aminos, or water along with herbs and spices to flavor your food. Your body has a hard time digesting oil. It clogs and congests the body; some oils are estrogenic and cause fibroids to grow especially soy oil. It is acid-forming, mucus forming, a hormone-disruptor, toxic, carcinogenic, and causes fibroids to grow.

Other misc. plant foods to avoid because in some women they cause symptoms to increase: Cashews, chickpeas or garbanzo beans, sesame seeds (white), white tahini, and flax seeds.

High Oestrogen Plant Foods - Some plant foods have high estrogen levels. These oestrogens are called phytoestrogens. Some of them like soybeans are no's because they cause too many issues in some women.

FOODS YOU CAN EAT WHEN YOU'RE TRYING TO SHRINK FIBROIDS NATURALLY

Water - Drinking plenty of water first thing in the morning and before every meal will help speed up detoxification (8 - 10 glasses everyday). Water also ensures your hormone levels are balanced at all times. You can spice it up with lemon for additional benefits.

Green Tea - Green tea is full of antioxidants. One **study** found that epigallocatechin gallate, an antioxidant found in green tea, fights inflammation and reduces high estrogen levels. This, in turn, reduces fibroid growth and blood loss. So start drinking green tea, if you haven't started already.

Beta-Carotene Rich Foods - Beta-carotene is an antioxidant that converts into vitamin A in the body. A diet rich in beta-carotene helps promote fertility and prevent fibroid growth. Food sources of beta-carotene include:
- Sweet potatoes
- Carrots
- Broccoli
- Leafy greens like spinach and kale
- Cantaloupe
- Red and yellow peppers
- Apricots

Potassium Rich Foods - Foods rich in potassium will help lower blood pressure and reduce fibroid growth. Examples of potassium-rich foods include:
- Bananas
- Citrus fruits
- Avocado
- Cantaloupe
- Collard greens
- Dates
- Lentils
- Oat bran
- Potatoes
- Tomatoes

Vitamin D Rich Foods - Vitamin D can be easily gotten from the sun, but if you're black and live in cooler climates, you may be at risk for a deficiency. **One study** showed that fibroid size correlated inversely with serum vitamin D levels in African American women. This means that vitamin D deficiency increases the growth of the fibroid. Examples of food that are rich in vitamin-D include:
- Cod liver oil
- Fortified whole-grain cereal
- Egg yolks

- Fatty fish
- Fortified juice

Poultry - Chicken and turkey are great alternatives to red meat for anyone with fibroids. They are rich in protein and do not contain oestrogens. However, always remember to go for organic meat products and trim off excess fats before cooking.

Fatty Fish - Fatty fish contain omega-3-fatty acids that help fight inflammation that could contribute to fibroid growth. Salmon, tuna, and mackerel are good examples of fishes that you should add to your diet.

Beans and Legumes - Beans and legumes contain a type of dietary fiber called soluble fiber. This type of fiber prevents spikes in blood sugar, aids weight loss, and slows the growth of fibroids. **Studies** also show that fiber may help to increase the fecal excretion of estrogen, which may reduce its levels in the body.

Whole Grains - Whole grains like oats, fonio, whole wheat, millet, teff, quinoa, and sorghum are rich in dietary fiber. Dietary fiber improves satiety, reduces constipation, and helps you lose weight.

Cruciferous Vegetables - Cruciferous vegetables like Broccoli, cauliflower, cabbage, kale, collard greens, brussel sprouts, Chinese cabbage, radishes, turnips, kohlrabi, rocket (arugula), watercress, and daikon and lettuce are examples of cruciferous vegetables you should be eating because they're loaded with dietary fiber and antioxidants.

Their high fiber content helps to cleanse out your colon, removing toxins and excess estrogen. One human **study** showed that indole-3-carbinol found in cruciferous vegetables reduced the activity of oestrogens in the body.

Green Leafy Vegetables - Green leafy vegetables contain flavonoids and other phytochemicals that act as antioxidants. Antioxidants are chemical-like substances that help our body fight disease-causing free radicals. These chemicals are abundant in spinach, pumpkin leaves, jute, and greens.

Citrus Fruits - Citrus fruits are full of antioxidants and phytochemicals that help prevent fibroid growth. **One study** revealed that women who consume citrus fruits are less likely to develop fibroids. So start loading up on citrus fruits today!

Flaxseed - This is a plant-based food that provides healthful fat, antioxidants and fiber. It contains lots of fibroid healing properties including phytoestrogens that help to replace harmful oestrogens produced naturally by the body. This way, flaxseed thwarts estrogen dominance, which facilitates growth of fibroids in the body.

Garlic and Onions - If you really want to shrink fibroids in your uterus, then begin to consume onions and garlic. Both are rich sources of antioxidants, which help to combat free radical damage to health cells in the body system including the pelvic region.
With constant consumption of these herbs, you're shutting the door against damage from free radicals — which could increase risk of developing a number of health conditions including fibroids — in your body.

Cold Water Fish - Deep sea cold-water fish such as salmon, sardines, tuna, and mackerel should be part of your diet to shrink fibroids. You may want to ask me why. The reason is simple: they are a rich source of essential fatty acids which are anti-inflammatory and can help promote hormone balance.

Eggs - Eggs, as you know, are a great source of protein. But there's more to protein with eggs from organically raised birds. This is because the diet of such birds are usually supplemented with essential fatty acids which consequently help them to produce eggs that are rich in omega-3 fatty acids needed for good health. Omega-3 fatty acids alongside vitamin B, vitamin E and magnesium are good for reducing symptoms of fibroids

DETOXIFY YOUR BODY AS AT WHEN NEEDED

This is the most important step to shrink fibroids. The liver is the body's largest gland. One of its major functions is to detoxify the entire body. If the liver is not working properly, the body will be filled with toxins and excess hormones estrogen is metabolized in the liver.

Estrogen that is not metabolized by the liver will continue to circulate and exert its effect on the body. Herbs that detoxify and strengthen the liver will help speed up the removal of excess estrogen, toxins and other impurities from the body.

To cleanse and strengthen the liver, these are the things you should do. Herbal cleansing to clear the gastrointestinal tract and fortify the liver:

One of the best herbs to fortify the liver is silymarin, a special extract of milk thistle. Others include: dandelion leaf and root, turmeric and artichoke.

21 HERBAL TEAS THAT WILL SHRINK YOUR FIBROIDS AND OVARIAN CYSTS

- Aidan fruit
- Negro pepper
- Piper Guineense
- Turmeric
- Ginger
- Garlic
- Cinnamon
- Nettle leaf
- Burdock root
- Chickweed
- Oregon grape fruit
- Dandelion root
- Red raspberry leaf
- Chaste tree leaf
- Red clover
- Maca root/powder
- Green tea
- Motherwort
- Flax seeds, chia seeds and hemp seeds
- Matcha tea
- Milk thistle

Make tea with any of the herbs and drink a cup on an empty stomach every morning. Making tea with them is that simple and easy. Boil water and a certain amount of the herbs with the water. Allow it to infuse for a few minutes, sieve and drink.

12 KEY SUCCESSES TO SHRINK FIBROIDS AND OVARIAN CYSTS

1. Avoid foods that increases the level of estrogen because estrogen is one of the major hormone that keeps fibroid growing bigger

2. Avoid soft drinks, industrial drinks, caffeinated drinks, and all drinks that has to do with soy products
3. Avoid eating refined sugars, carbohydrate sugars, and alcoholic drinks
4. Avoid fatty foods, foods high in salt and diary drinks
5. Avoid melon soups
6. Eat cruciferous vegetables like lettuces, cabbage, broccoli, watercress or water leaf, cauliflower, Brussels sprouts, kale etc, all these vegetables are rich in vitamins such as Vitamins C, K, B2, B6 and folic acid, which is very good for womens' health.
7. Ensure you eat beans daily.
8. Drink natural juices, smoothies and drinks that helps to heal fibroids everyday
9. Eat vegetable salads
10. Drink lots of water at least a minimum of 8 glasses of water daily.
11. Eat only natural and local foods. Ensure you avoid all flour made foods such as cakes, pastries, cookies, snacks, etc.
12. Take some women's multivitamins like Vitabiotics wellwoman max, Vitamin D supplement, potassium supplements, omega 3 fatty acids etc.

CHAPTER THREE

MY FIBROID AND CYSTS JOURNEY STORY

My name is Favour Marius, the founder of <u>Natural Health Remedies</u> Facebook page.

I am a young and vibrant woman of our time like you. I am a natural health enthusiast

I am here to share with you my fibroid and cysts journey story and why I have decided in my heart to journey down through the path of herbs and natural remedies.

Me and my family are a living testimony of what diets, herbs and spices can do to someone. In the year 2018 to 2021 I nearly lost one of my ovaries (left ovary) but God of Creation, who has given us these herbs said NO.

Today I am healed and made whole through herbs. I no longer cry of pain. I have been certified free. No more fibroid, ovarian cysts and fibroadenosis.

It was only diets, herbs and spices I used after the hospital failed me and I am free.

Indeed there is power in these herbs. No wonder Christian Bible said in the book of Genesis that God has given us these herbs to be our food and medicine.

But we humans, we disregard it and pursue pharmaceutical medicines. The truth is that sometimes these pharmaceutical medicines fail us.

Therefore, since I have got this miracle through herbs, and I know there are many women out there going through the same pain I went through.

Some have not even been able to get pregnant after their marriage due to the same monsters called fibroid and ovarian cyst.

That's why I have created this book and WhatsApp group to share my story, herbal remedies and also support my fellow women to gain their freedom from fibroids and ovarian cysts.

My story in details . . .

In February 2018, I was diagnosed with a simple ovarian cyst on my left. After the whole ultrasound scan, my gynecologist gave me some medication and assured me that I will be fine.

The truth is that after I took the medication, the pain subsided. I was happy again with my life and cruising life with the hope that I am free.

Not until November 2018 (that's exactly 9 months after the first scan), I was struck with this intense and chronic pelvic pain that kept me crying all day.

I can't sit comfortably, I can't stand comfortably and I can't lay down comfortably. I was miserable and got tired of life.

I had to visit my gynecologist again. Another ultrasound scan was conducted on me. And the result came out with "complex ovarian cyst and anterior Intramural uterine leiomyoma (uterine fibroids)."

I fainted! At what age . . . No, I am very young for this kind of sickness and no one in my family both immediate and extended has had such diseases or infections. Why me?

I began asking questions, doctor, what is the cause of fibroid and ovarian cyst? Do they not have a cure?

My gynecologist looked at me eye to eyeball and told me that there's no cure for fibroid and ovarian cyst except surgery.

There are no causes for now but there are risk factors that trigger such infections like family history, hormonal imbalance, consuming junks and fast foods, soft drinks, industrial drinks, miscarriage, etc.

My eyes opened wide and my jaw dropped. Doctor, what is the solution? All I want now is a solution to come out of pain, is too much for me.

We will be giving you some medication and painkillers to help you manage the pains.

We will keep monitoring the growth. If it goes to the extreme, we have to remove them. Fear gripped me because I have this phobia of going under the knife (surgery).

I quickly went to the pharmaceutical shop close to the hospital. That was where I discovered that the drugs that were prescribed for me were the same drugs I took earlier without result (it moved from simple to complex).

This is when I knew that I am on my own, if I don't act quickly I will end up going for surgery and I may lose my left ovary. I left the pharmacy to my house without those medications.

During this period, one thing kept my faith, which is 'I believe that there's a solution to every problem on earth except death' but since I am not dead but alive, then I should be able to get a solution to these two infections (fibroid and ovarian cyst).

I believe a solution is somewhere and I had to find it.

I got myself soaked in research. I began to research every herb and spice in the world, preparing them and taking them.

While I was researching how to drive my healing myself, I went into fasting so that the fibroid won't keep growing, I was afraid of surgery. I ate once daily.

I kept fasting and doing daily exercise every morning. Once I wake up from bed, I will pick up my rope and start skipping. I started with 50 counts daily and graduated to 100 counts. I do this rope skipping every morning.

I also eat once a day. My food then was only beans, sweet potatoes, fruits and plenty of vegetables until I discovered these herbal solutions that I prepared that hasten my healing. I mean total healing.

I prepared a lot of remedies that I took and I also charted a new diet plan for myself. I became my own herbal doctor and nutritionist.

God of Creation really gave me victory. I have these remedies in the chapter four section of this book.

I started with number 7 remedy because that was the first remedy I discovered by trial and error, I noticed that the pain of ovarian cysts has reduced drastically. After the first 30 days of drinking remedy number I discovered number 3.

The number 3 worked well on my fibroid size. While I was taking the number 3 remedy I discovered a higher recipe to modify the number 3 remedy. That was how I came up with the **number one remedy**. Boom, the fibroid began to shrink and finally shrunk.

I also took smoothies, teas and many other things. But the ones written in this book are the real deal.

As I was treating fibroid and ovarian cyst, in August 2019, I was diagnosed with a massive lump in my two breasts (the medical name for infection is FIBROADENOSIS). Problem became too much for me. It was a serious burden to take off my shoulders.

Finally I got a solution that shrinks fibroid, ovarian cyst and fibroadenosis naturally without surgery. Hallelujah! My fibroadenosis healing is a story from another book.

Smile and laugh that came out of my innermost heart that day I went for the last ultrasound scan and I was declared healed - it was from a very pure and joyous heart.

I quote the doctor " young woman you can go home now, everything is fine. Your pelvic scan is clean and clear. Nothing was found there anymore".

Oh my God, I am so happy and excited today telling you my life story as a young woman of 33 years old and how I was able to find a solution to my problem myself.

These herbs are amazing. They are powerful and offer total healing from the root.

The journey of my healing was not easy. I must confess that. It took me determination, daily positive affirmations, strict and continuous usage of my new diet plan and remedies to achieve my goal, which is total healing from fibroid, ovarian cyst and fibroadenosis.

I want to assure you, no matter what problem you're passing through today, there's a solution to it.

Finally, if you have decided to heal yourself using herbs, spices and foods as medicine? Then you have to wear patience and determination like cloth. Because healing with herbs is slow but cures ultimately from root.

I sincerely thank you for purchasing this book. My hope is that as you consistently consume the recipes contained on these pages, you will see changes in your body quickly.

May the God of Creation bless you and grant you genuine and lasting healing both physically, emotionally and spiritually.

If you have questions or need further assistance, please send me an email at diyhomemaderecipes@gmail.com, **makafavour@gmail.com**, or follow my facebook page here.

I am hoping and praying for your complete and total healing for your mind, body, and soul.

Many blessings to you!

CHAPTER FOUR

These are herbal remedies I used to heal myself. If you follow these remedies strictly with my guide, be sure you'll get positive results within 3 months to 12 months depending on the size of your fibroids and cysts.

These natural remedies are very effective and it yields results. I am not writing hearsay remedies but I am giving you remedies that I used myself and it worked for me and today I am very happy that I discovered them.

Without much ado, let's dive in immediately!

SEVEN HERBAL SOLUTIONS FOR HEALING FIBROIDS AND OVARIAN CYSTS

The herbs for these solutions are powerful and have been proven to eliminate fibroid and other female reproductive related problems. Though the herbs are mostly common in Africa but can be found in other parts of the world.

These are used in my country Nigeria (Eastern part of Nigeria) to cook for a postpartum mum for the first month of her delivery. What is the work of these herbs in her?

The herbs and spices have been put in her food to help flush out any unwanted substances or bad blood remaining on her uterus and to prevent her from having any female reproductive related problems like fibroid, blocked fallopian tube, cysts, endometriosis, PCOS etc.

And these have been for us over.

So I urge you to please take this remedy seriously so you can get the result you're looking for:

- Aidan fruit [Tetrapleura Tetraptera]
- Negro pepper
- Piper guineense
- Cloves
- Ginger
- Garlic
- Guava leaves
- Mango inner seed
- Turmeric

- Maca root
- Avocado seed
- Lemon pineapple peel etc.

Note you're not to take all the remedies at the same time. Choose one of the remedies from number 1 to 5 if your problem is fibroid and stick to it for like 30 days before you can change to another remedy if you wish.

If yours is ovarian cyst, choose any of the remedies from number 4, 6 and 7, however you can also use any of the number 1 to 5 remedies.

Then if you're suffering from blocked fallopian tube, use number 3 remedies continuously, you will get results:

Recipes Number One

- Aidan fruit - 3 pieces
- Garlic - 2 bulbs
- Ginger - enough quantity
- Cinnamon sticks - 3 pieces
- Negro pepper - 5 sticks
- Piper guineense - 1 teaspoon
- Water - 5 liters

Direction:
1. Cut Aidan fruit into three pieces each and put in a clean pot, fill the pot with 5 liters of water.
2. Cut every other ingredient into smaller pieces and add also into the pot.
3. Allow it to boil for 30 to 45 minutes and bring it down to cool a little. Drink while it's still hot 3 times daily.

Dosage:
- Drink a glass this remedy on empty stomach in the morning 30 minutes before breakfast
- Drink a glass 2 hours before lunch
- A glass cup at night, last thing to bed.

Note: If your fibroid is big, then do this exercise after drinking this remedy each time.

After drinking this remedy in the morning or afternoon or evening, go back to your bed and lay down as if you want to push out a baby, then continue to massage your tummy for like 10 to 15 minutes, get up and go about your normal duties.

Ensure to do this each time you take the remedy until you're declared free by a sonographer.

Recipe Number Two

- 5 Aidan stick
- 5 avocado seed
- 30 mango inner seed
- 50 soursop leaves
- 50 guava leaves
- Two handful of ginger
- Two bulb garlic
- Unripe papaya or the leaves
- 5 liters of water

Direction:

1. Cut the Aidan sticks and put first inside the pot
2. Cut the avocado seeds and mango seeds ,ginger, garlic and add to the pot.
3. If you have beetroot add it as well.
4. Then put in the soursop leaves and papaya leaves.
5. Add pap water or normal water to cook for 20 to 30 minutes. Bring it down to cool a little and drink twice a day (morning and night) while it's hot.

Dosage:

- Drink a glass in the morning on empty stomach 20 minutes before breakfast and last thing to bed at night after dinner

Note: While drinking the medicine avoid food that is not friendly with fibroid then drink this medicine for four weeks and go for Scan.

If the fibroid was too big it must have reduced then continue drinking to completely eliminate it from your system.

If it's a small fibroid, it must have disappeared after four weeks.

Recipe Number Three

- 2 sticks of Aidan fruit
- 10 sticks of Negro pepper
- A teaspoon of Piper guineense
- A pinch of salt
- 4 liters of water

Directions:

1. Cut and boil two sticks of Aidan fruit into small pieces, with ten sticks of Uda, and a teaspoon of Negro pepper using four litres of water. Add a pinch of salt.
2. Drink while hot, two shots morning and night (Before menses and during menses).

Dosage:

- Drink a glass this remedy on empty stomach in the morning 30 minutes before breakfast
- Drink a glass 2 hours before lunch
- A glass cup at night, last thing to bed.

Recipe Number Four
- Aidan fruit - 3 pieces
- Fresh lemon - 2
- Fresh pineapple peels (skin) - enough quantity
- Cloves - one cup
- Negro pepper - 3 pieces
- Water - 3 liters

Direction:

1. Cut Aidan fruit, lemon and negro pepper into smaller pieces add inside pot and add all other ingredients together with 3 liters of water and boil for 25 to 30 minutes.
2. Bring it down to cool a little and drink it hot twice daily.

Dosage:

- Drink a glass on empty stomach 30 minutes before breakfast and last thing to bed at night after dinner.

Recipe Number Five

- Guava leaves - 30 leaves
- Soursop leaves - 30 leaves
- Aidan fruit - 3 sticks
- Cloves - one cup
- Ginger - enough quantity
- Cinnamon - 3 sticks
- Water - 5 liters

Direction:

1. Cut Aidan fruit into three pieces, add it with every other ingredient to a pot, add water and boil for 30 mins.
2. Bring it down to cool and drink twice a day for as long as needed until your fibroids or cysts are gone

Dosage:

- Take half glass on an empty stomach 20 to 30 minutes before breakfast and last thing to bed at night after dinner.

Recipe Number Six

- A handful fresh Ginger
- One bulb Garlic
- One and half handful fresh Turmeric
- 2 tablespoon Cloves
- One big Maca root
- 2 liters of water

Direction:

1. Wash and peel the back of the garlic, ginger, turmeric and maca roots and dice into pieces.
2. Wash the cloves and add to the ingredients also.
3. Then soak all the ingredients together with water in an empty container for minimum of 48 hours, maximum of 72 hours (i.e 2 to 3 days)
4. After 3 days, sieve the mixture to remove the herbs inside the bottle to avoid them getting decayed.

5. After sieving preserve the tea or juice inside the bottle. Store in a refrigerator or under room temperature if you don't refrigerator.

Dosage:

- Take half a glass of this maca combo on empty stomach first thing in the morning before meals and last thing at night before bed.

NB: Take as long as you feel the need to

Those that can take it:
- Men and women can take it.
- Children above the ages of 16
- Singles can take it (unmarried).
- Trying to conceive mums
- Couples wanting to boost their sexual Libido.

Caution:

- If you're trying to conceive, DO NOT take during your ovulation and most especially your fertile days. The best time for those wanting to conceive is while Menstruating.
- Do not take it when you are not sure if you're already pregnant.
- Not to be taken by pregnant and nursing mothers.
- Not to be taken while on drugs or other medications.
- Not to be taken if you have Ulcer, some of the ingredients will trigger the ulcer and aggravate it.
- If you are allergic to any of the herbs in the mixture, kindly STOP using immediately.

Recipe Number Seven

- 1½ handful of fresh turmeric root
- 1 handful fresh ginger root
- 1 bulb raw garlic (fresh)
- 2 tablespoon cloves
- 1.5litres water
- Container for storage

Method of Preparation:

1. Peel off the skin of turmeric, ginger and garlic, wash them clean and grate them together or cut them into small pieces with a knife. But I prefer to pound it with mortar.
2. After grating, add them into the empty container you have for storage.
3. Wash clove pods and add it into the container, add 1.5 liters of water into it, cover with lid and keep it where it will not be disturbed under room temperature for 3 days to ferment.
4. After 3 days, bring it out, sieve it and throw away the chaff. Then return the juice into the bottle and cover.
5. Start taking it every morning and night.

Dosage:

- Take ½ glass of turmeric and ginger combo in an empty stomach in the morning 30 minutes before meal and last thing to bed at night after dinner.

Note For All Remedies Listed Above
- Follow all procedures strictly as stated.
- While taking these remedies avoid everything you suppose to avoid, anything that grows fibroids and cysts, you must avoid it if you want this recipe to work for you.
- Do not take all the remedies at once. Choose one of the remedies each month and prepare. What I mean is use one of the remedies each month until your Ultrasound Scan says there are no traces of fibroids or cysts again.
- These remedies also work for all kinds of female infections and PIDs
- All cooked or boiled remedies must be taken when it's hot please. On no account should you drink it cold.

Caution:

If your problem is only infections and you're trying to conceive please take these remedies only when you're menstruating to avoid miscarrying your baby especially number six and seven remedies.

CHAPTER FIVE

Everything I am sharing in this book is all I used to heal myself from fibroids and ovarian Cysts, please take them seriously if you really want healing.

SMOOTHIES AND JUICES FOR HEALING FIBROIDS AND OVARIAN CYSTS

1. Pineapple Smoothie

- 1 large pineapple
- 1 medium beetroot
- A thumb size ginger

Direction:

1. In a basin of water containing water and white vinegar, soak the 3 beets with the leaves for 2 to 3 minutes.
2. Rinse them well under running water.
3. Peel the pineapple skin and cut into chunks.
4. Remove the leaves of the beets then cut the beets into chunks also, throw all ingredients including the beet leaves into a blender and blend until smooth. Or if you prefer juice over smoothie you can use your juicer to juice them.
5. Enjoy on an empty stomach 20 minutes before breakfast.

2. Apple Carrot Juice

- 5 small Apples
- 7 medium carrots
- A thumb size ginger

Direction:

1. Juice them and store in a refrigerator.
2. Take ½ glass morning, afternoon and night daily.

NB: If you don't have juicer you can use your blender.

3. Berries Smoothie
- 1 cup coconut water
- ½ cup mixed berries (strawberries & blueberries)
- ½ banana
- ½ cup almond milk
- Shredded coconut for dressing

Direction:

1. Throw into a blender all ingredients and blend until smooth. Serve in a glass and top up with shredded coconut.
2. Enjoy on an empty stomach 20 minutes before breakfast and 1 hour before dinner

4. Celery Lettuce Smoothie (Alkaline Juice)
- 2 heads Celery
- 2 heads lettuce
- 1 large cucumber
- 4 lemon fruit (peeled.and segmented)
- 5 cups mixed greens (packed)
- ½ cup water or any nut milk of your choice

Direction:

1. Add all ingredients into the juicer and serve or store for up to 3 days in a glass jar in the refrigerator.

5. Apple Beet Juice
- 8 red Apples
- 2 medium beetroots
- 1 cup almond milk

Direction:

1. Add all ingredients into the juicer and serve
2. Drink this apple and beets juice 4 cups daily for maximum result.

6. Cabbage Smoothie
- 1 head green cabbage
- 2 green Apples
- 1 whole lemon
- 1 cup filtered water

Direction:

1. Wash and cut all ingredients into chunks, throw into a blender and blend until smooth.
2. Enjoy on an empty stomach 20 minutes before breakfast.

7. Coconut Mango Smoothie
- 1 cup coconut water
- ½ cup mango chunks
- ½ banana
- 1 inch ginger or 1 tsp. ginger powder
- 1 tablespoon pure coconut oil
- 3 inches turmeric root
- 2 pinches cinnamon powder
- 1 teaspoon flax seeds or chia seeds

Direction:

1. Throw all ingredients into a blender and blend until smooth.
2. Enjoy on an empty stomach 20 minutes before breakfast.

It can even serve as a meal replacement. So feel free to use morning and night as a meal replacement.

8. Pear Mango Smoothie
- 2 Pears
- 2 cups Mango chunks
- 2 tbsp. ginger powder
- 1inch turmeric root
- 4 tablespoon sea moss gel
- 1 tsp. ground cinnamon
- 1 banana

- 3 medjool dates
- ½ cup coconut milk
- 2½ cups filtered water

Direction:

1. Add all ingredients into a blender and blend until smooth.
2. Enjoy on an empty stomach 20 minutes before breakfast.

9. Cucumber Apple Smoothie
- 2 bunches Celery
- 2 large cucumber
- 1 medium beet
- 3 small Apple
- 3 small chunks of turmeric
- 1 inch ginger
- 2 whole lemon (peeled)
- ½ jalapeno
- 1 spring of fresh mint
- ½ small bunch Dandelion greens
- 2 cups spinach (packed)

Direction:

1. Cut ingredients to fit your juicer. Run ingredients through your juicer. Serve or store in glass airtight jars for up to 3 days.
2. Enjoy on an empty stomach 20 minutes before breakfast.

10. Spinach Banana Smoothie
- 5 to 6 cups of baby spinach
- 2 big ripen bananas
- 1 tsp. ground turmeric
- 1 tsp. spirulina powder
- 1 tsp. barley grass powder
- 1 tsp. wheatgrass powder
- Dragon fruit
- Mixed berries
- 1 cup filtered water

Direction:

1. Add all ingredients into a blender and blend until smooth.
2. Enjoy on an empty stomach 20 minutes before breakfast.

NATURAL DRINKS FOR HEALING FIBROIDS AND OVARIAN CYSTS

Drink A
- 1 tbsp. blackstrap molasses (unsulphured)
- 1 tbsp. Apple cider vinegar
- 1 whole lemon (juiced)
- 1 tbsp. aluminum free pure baking soda (optional)

Direction:

1. Add all ingredients in glass and dilute with a ½ glass warm water

Dosage:

- Drink this morning, afternoon and night

Drink B.
- 61/4 cups filtered water
- 1 cup hemp seeds
- 2 thumb turmeric
- 4 pitted Dates (optional)

Direction:

1. Add all the ingredients in the blender and blend until smooth.
2. Strain the liquid to separate the pump from the milk.
3. Store in the refrigerator and consume within three days.

Dosage:

- Drink morning, afternoon and night daily

Drink C.

- 1 cup Apple cider vinegar
- ½ cup Blackstrap molasses
- 7 Oranges
- 1 bulb Garlic
- ¼ cup pure Honey
- 3 Beetroots
- 25g fresh ginger

Direction:

1. Mix all ingredients inside a glass jar.
2. Take about 40ml of the mixture into a drinking glass and mix with warm water. Drink three times daily

Drink D

- 1 tbsp Apple cider vinegar
- 1 tbsp blackstrap molasses
- 1 glass of warm filtered water

Direction:

1. Add apple cider vinegar into a glass of warm water
2. Add blackstrap molasses and mix them together. You can store it in the refrigerator for three days.

Dosage:

- Drink one to two glasses daily.

ANTI INFLAMMATORY TEAS AND SMOOTHIES

Drink A

- 1 cup fresh ginger
- 1 cup fresh turmeric
- 1 whole lemon (juiced)

- 2 tablespoons honey
- 4 liters of coconut water
- A dash of black pepper

Direction:

1. Blend all ingredients together with a blender. Pour into a pot to bring to a boil, turn off the heat and allow it to simmer for 20 minutes while the pot is still covered.
2. Add a juice of one lemon and 2 tablespoons of honey or blackstrap molasses, or date paste/syrup and stir together.
3. After stirring all together, strain out the juice. Pour in an airtight container/bottle and store in a refrigerator.

Dosage:

- Drink one glass of turmeric tea every morning. You can garnish with a lemon wedge.

Drink B.
- 1 ginger
- A dash of cayenne pepper
- ¼ cup coconut water.

Direction:

- Blend all together, strain into a glass and enjoy!

Drink C.
- 1 tablespoon fresh grated turmeric
- 1 teaspoon fresh grated ginger
- 1 cup nut milk
- 2 cups of pineapple chunks
- 1 ripe banana

Direction:

1. Blend all together, and enjoy!

Drink D.
- 2 cups coconut water
- 2 cups of blueberries
- 1 ripe banana
- ½ cup of Greek yogurt
- 1 tablespoon flaxseed

Direction:

1. Blend all together, and enjoy!

Drink E.
- 3 medium size carrot, peeled and cut into chunks
- 1 medium beets
- 1 orange (juiced)
- 1 thumb size ginger
- 1 cup filtered water

Direction:

1. Blend all together, strain into a glass and enjoy!

Drink F.
- 1 lime (juice)
- 3 celery sticks
- 2 big red apple
- 1 cucumber
- 3 kale leaves
- 1 handful spinach

Direction:

1. Blend all together, strain into a glass and enjoy!

POWERFUL HORMONE BALANCING SMOOTHIES

Smoothie one

- 1 cup unsweetened almond milk
- ½ cup frozen banana
- 1 cup avocado
- A handful spinach
- 1 stalk celery
- 2 tablespoon ground chia seed
- 1 tablespoon fresh lemon juice
- 1 teaspoon ashwagandha powder
- 1 teaspoon maca powder

Direction:

1. Blend all together and enjoy!

Smoothie Two
- 1 cup unsweetened almond milk
- A handful spinach
- ½ cup frozen banana
- 1 cup avocado
- 1 tbsp. hemp seeds
- 1 tbsp. almond butter
- 1 tbsp. cocoa powder
- 1 teaspoon maca powder

Direction:

1. Blend all together and enjoy!

Smoothie Three

- 1 cup unsweetened almond milk
- 2 handful spinach
- ½ cup frozen strawberries
- ½ cup frozen raspberries
- 1 teaspoon ashwagandha powder

- 2 tablespoon ground chia seeds
- 1 tablespoon of flaxseed oil

Direction:

1. Blend all together and enjoy!

Smoothie Four
- ½ cup frozen Zucchini
- 1 cup organic spinach
- ½ cup organic green grapes
- 1 dates
- 1 tablespoon almond butter
- 1 cup nut milk
- ½ teaspoon Cinnamon powder.

Direction:

1. Blend all together and enjoy!

HERBS IMAGES FOR EASY RECOGNITION

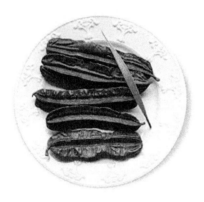

TETRAPLEURA TETRAPTERA (AIDAN FRUIT)

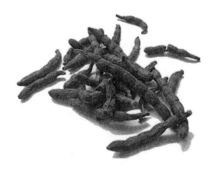

NEGRO PEPPER

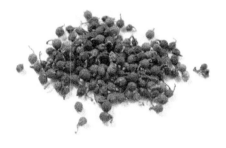

PIPER GUINEENSE (please this is not black peppercorn)

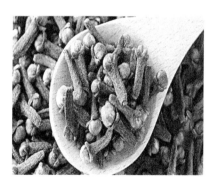

CLOVES

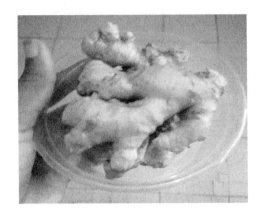

GINGER

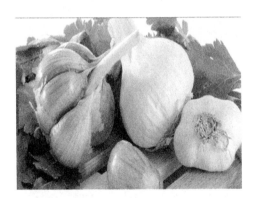

GARLIC

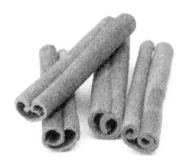

CINNAMON STICKS

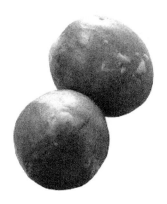

AVOCADO SEED

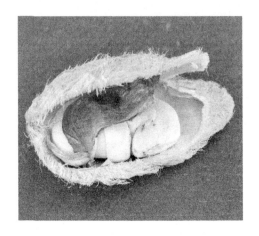

MANGO INNER SEED

Printed in Great Britain
by Amazon